The Boneheap in the Lion's Den

THE BONEHEAP IN THE LION'S DEN

Winner of the Press 53 Award for Poetry

MAYA J. SORINI

Press 53
Winston-Salem

Press 53, LLC
PO Box 30314
Winston-Salem, NC 27130

First Edition

A Tom Lombardo Poetry Selection

The Boneheap in the Lion's Den
Winner of the 2023 Press 53 Award for Poetry

Cover art licensed through iStock

Cover design by Kevin Morgan Watson

Library of Congress Control Number
2023932020

ISBN 978-1-950413-60-7

For my patients

Contents

Moratorium

Say what you mean.
Stop saying "expired"
Like it is inevitable for the 28-year-old
To die on a Tuesday at noon.

Stop keeping it a few words away from you,
Using "expired" because "death" forces
You to think about
Your grandfather's funeral
When you were 16 and had never seen
Your dad cry before.

Say what you mean exactly—
Do not say, "we did everything we could"
When what you mean is
"I have given every tear and deep breath I have to this job
But the bullets keep winning.
I don't want to be
The one telling you
That we lose every
Day to scraps of metal."

Say what you really mean:
"Your son is dead."

Cardiomegaly

Who told the heart it could be so small, who made us grow proportional to it, why aren't we just hearts beating around, could have added more chambers, made the whole body pulse alive, we are alive, aren't we? Who's to say we shouldn't twitch in the petri dish? Who decided to let some of our cells rest while others have to push-pull all the time? I guess I still avoid talking about him, the dead man whose heart I held, warm from his body, so recently dead, the trauma surgeon in a callous teaching moment let us touch inside his chest, let us hold his heart, still twitching from epinephrine injections, warm and heavy, soft as a kitten, trying to make him live.

Red

My mother's favorite color
The ruby glass she collects
Makes patterned prisms
The azaleas behind the fence
A scratched mosquito bite
The lights on ambulances
Hit by truck drizzling the floor
An exposed strawberry ice cream belly
With hands inside throwing man overboard
Clots and shit splattering floor
Up to our knees stained

Rate Your Pain:

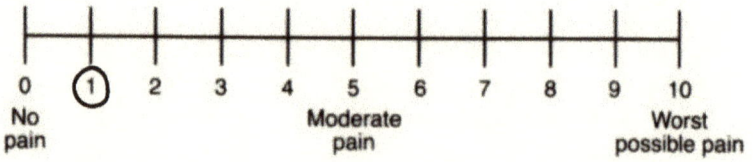

```
   |  |  |  |  |  |  |  |  |  |  |
   0 (1) 2  3  4  5  6  7  8  9  10
  No               Moderate        Worst
  pain               pain      possible pain
```

the clickpopsssssstt of an opening can

The Body Only Speaks Her Own Language

The body cannot make sense of bullet's ricochet from pelvis up through bowels and back off rib, and will not apologize. The body doesn't speak lead, she speaks blood, knowing so well its pulse that upon introduction of mechanical pump to replace arrhythmic heart, the body rebels, pushing insidious blood into intestines whisper by whisper. The body only speaks her native language. She does not compromise, will not be colonized, cannot be forced to assimilate to our messy, inexact tongues. She bleeds. She knows how to do this. She does it expertly. We say, "rate your pain?" but her retort is electric and sticky with blood, impossible to translate, even when you have thrown your life at the task of decoding her messages. My heartbeat is a tinnitus, a ringing through my body, I do not get to ignore it. Sometimes we manage to communicate in a pidgin of our languages, hanging on each other's every word, using every ounce of energy we have to speak. These days I am poring over dictionaries, bleeding into google translate, trying to find an interpreter so that when she uses words I don't understand, someone can help me put together more sentences. I need to get this much across: Dear body, be brave.

Hurting Instructions

Remind your shaking voice that scrapes heal faster than bruises heal faster than bones heal faster than the feeling that the screech of metal will finish your sentences and the and the sensation of sudden acceleration towards and the feeling the feeling of blood warm down your face as you crawl out of car onto ground and apologize for bleeding into it. Wake up and take your whatever your you can get your your mine hands on and touch your— the face that is yours only because it was grandfathered in touch your nose that was numb after— when you were on the ground seeping when—my words won't come out right— I have torn down the lost posters and spit out the pills. There are parts of me that will never come home.

Massive Transfusion Protocol

Then there was nothing but blood, pint after pint after pint after pint
after pint after pint after pint after pint after pint after pint after pint
after pint after pint after pint after pint after pint after pint after pint
after pint after pint after pint after pint after pint after pint after pint
after pint after pint after pint after pint after pint after pint after pint
after pint after pint after pint after pint after pint after pint after pint
after pint after pint after pint after pint after pint after pint after pint
after pint after pint after pint after pint after pint after pint after pint
after pint after pint after pint after pint after pint after pint after pint
after pint after pint after pint after pint after pint after pint after pint
after pint after pint after pint after pint after pint after pint after pint
after pint after pint after pint after pint after pint after pint after pint
after pint after pint after pint after pint after pint after pint after pint
after pint after pint after pint after pint after pint after pint after pint
after pint after pint after pint after pint after pint after pint after pint
after pint after pint after pint after pint after pint after pint after pint
after pint after pint after pint after pint after pint after pint after pint
after pint after pint after pint after pint after pint after pint after pint
after pint after pint after pint after pint after pint after pint after pint
after pint after pint after pint after pint after pint after pint after pint
after pint after pint after pint after pint after pint after pint after pint
after pint after pint after pint after pint after pint after pint after pint
after pint after pint after pint after pint after pint after pint after pint
after pint after pint after pint after pint after pint after pint after pint
after pint after pint after pint after pint after pint after pint after pint
after pint after pint after pint after pint after pint after pint after pint
after pint after pint after pint after pint after pint after pint after pint
after pint after pint after pint after pint after pint after pint after pint
after pint after pint after pint after pint after pint after pint after pint
after pint after pint after pint after pint after pint after pint after pint
after pint after pint after pint after pint after pint after pint after pint
after pint after pint after pint after pint after pint after pint after pint
after pint after pint after pint after pint,

To replace his life force twenty-two-times over
Until there was none of him left

That Smell

I tell my Stop the Bleed students our goal is to keep blood in bodies by any means necessary I tell them I don't care if you don't have a tourniquet or gloves or gauze take the shirt off your back and stuff your fingers deep into the hot trench of bleeding until it stops Sometimes they worry about HIV or hepatitis and I try to remain neutral when repeating my assigned You have to keep yourself safe first. These students know nothing. Surely they have bitten their tongue and tasted blood, but they don't know it like I do. Blood doesn't smell by itself, it only smells when you put it up next to plastic The two of them compound each other and expire a ghost of both things: the inorganic rust of the iron spilling from the body with the organic artifice of a factory floor doused in turpentine It is the worst of all smells It will haunt you like a blended monster, a Chupacabra licking its soaked paws, waiting. I met the Chupacabra years ago, before the hospital's whitewash made him my unwilling colleague See I know something terrible but I can't tell the students I can't say You can try and keep yourself safe but every time I hold a reeking blood bag I remember being the only one brave enough to don dishwashing gloves and pick bloody condoms off the floor of a friend's bedroom as she slept on the couch instead of in her blood-soaked bed.

Rate Your Pain:

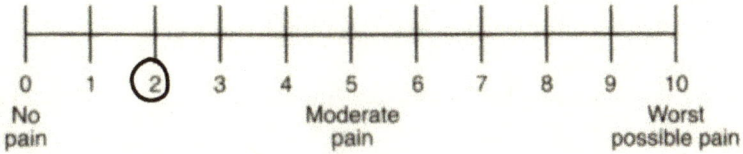

```
 |—|—|—|—|—|—|—|—|—|—|
 0   1  (2)  3   4   5   6   7   8   9   10
No                Moderate              Worst
pain                pain            possible pain
```

Just after you've bitten your tongue,

Something slimier, a remnant of primordial soup.

Eavesdropping on the Dead

Today I heard a man talk to his mother about her eulogy.
They decided on the color of her funeral flowers—
Purple, and white
He kept reminding her to swallow her water
And finished his sentences with "mama,"
So she would remember she was supposed to be listening.

I watched a woman brush the oily hair from her husband's forehead
She spoke like velvet,
Telling him how good he looked
With that tube sticking out of his mouth,
Sitting up today!

There is Arabic music playing down the hall
Because a patriarch is dying
Zaeem, Omar Almadani
Allah ateyk alf afyeeh
The family told the doctors they were so thankful for them.

The dead tell stories
They forget to swallow
They sign papers
That say they would like to die soon
They listen to music
They pick flowers
They have tubes in their mouths, in their arms, in their bellies,
They laugh and laugh and laugh

I Dreamed I Coughed Up My Spine

A V of wild geese broken, scattering the hard cold sky
I kept saying "help me"
On escalators and up stairs
Trying to hold my back together with open fingers
Not sure if I would suddenly become paralyzed
I kept yelling but
Nobody would
Help me

Summer Sinking

In the hours between dusk and dawn you will know the trip   fall
Pain of saying no not today.

Not   again   today.

Not   a   child   again   today .
Begging through your fingers
That somehow the hours will pass
The trees will shed
And the winter of closed doors and wet floors will save

Some of the children from each other's guns

How to Heal

Name a part of you that doesn't hurt.
Name it God.

Rate Your Pain:

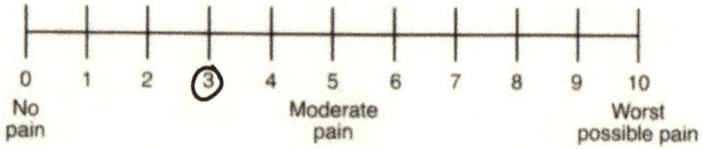

```
|  |  |  |  |  |  |  |  |  |  |
0  1  2  ③  4  5  6  7  8  9  10
No            Moderate        Worst
pain            pain       possible pain
```

Overgrown too closed
to the kidney spine snaggletooth

Of ick glossing the fish eyes.

Even When It Breaks

Kidney do not go eyes either nervy jump crackle find one mistake xeroxed by trillions teaching blame lungs avoiding greyness and light fizzle Euphrates saxophone starting to know pearls ready cherry blossom ova ovary overture ovation with extra lane and no off ramps irises leaking edge light worried beneath deadly ancient snow they secure blue skin trace my finger up forgetting bone cautery barbeque to watch pauses pooling shut up I realize I did not study history because it is drowning me.

The Lies

She died. She died in the bathroom, never reaching the phone from the tub, burning to death in an instant. She was never trapped for hours until EMS collected her. She never had her smoking body pushed through our emergency room, never made it smell like a firepit and burnt hair, never had a tube forced down her scorched throat, never had her skin peeled from her limbs, never was wrapped in cold wet gauze as she cried from the anguish, despite the sedation, despite the tube in her mouth. She never forgot how to breathe every morning, never had a tube sewn into her neck, never cried for weeks. She never painstakingly taught her skin to re-grow, all alone. She never brought me to my knees with grief, never sat with open eyes as I stroked her teary cheeks with my gloved thumb. No. She died in the fire, instantly, went up in a rush of cigarette smoke. Her daughters threw her a funeral with purple and white flowers. They sang "Amazing Grace" and "I'll Fly Away" and they cried together for many hours. She rests under the soft earth now, not crying out, never feeling any pain. She is not disfigured and scarred because she died in the fire. On the night of the burial, her daughters and their daughters stood by the grave, bellies still full of funeral fruit, celebrating the memory of how she had lived.

And Your Daughters Shall Prophesy

I dream of a man in the dark with a gun to a woman's head. I grab his arm and move the gun away and she has the look of the scream when there is a loud sound and the blood begins to spread. The hole in her shoulder from the small gun, handful of gun like a dead songbird, the small bullet makes a small hole red and wet her white shirt, the one she wore yesterday. Her face frozen, the man still holding the gun, the gun that is a baby's hand disappearing in his palm by the sink in the dark.

Rate Your Pain:

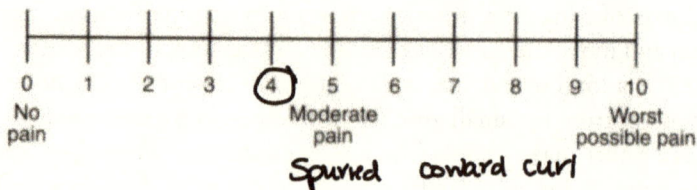

```
  0   1   2   3   4   5   6   7   8   9   10
 No             Moderate              Worst
pain              pain           possible pain
```

Spurred conward curl

Muscle up on bone

Making strange

the leg.

Caveat to Moratorium

Say what you mean, but
Do not make it about you.
Stop yourself from saying,
"Your son made me think of my first miscarriage,
Losing a child in a puddle of blood for no reason,
And I cried for three minutes in the bathroom
Before coming to break this news.
I loved your son because I loved mine,
And now they are gone.
I am sorry.
Our sons are dead."

St. Louis Sirens

Just like the rain, the heavy scent of asphalt precedes each large drop
hitting the black slick, measured in decibels or gallons to the gutter
textured air fleecing four o'clock motionless-less wet tumult dredging
down hot black light whips thunder through open fingers ringing the
maw of earth hungry to engulf to be eaten alive the glass gone molten
the best thing about bleeding is no matter what, it stops.

Chest X-Ray

That man I loved was in my dream again. He stood on my childhood lawn in deep night as the sound of peeping frogs and singing crickets poured through the woods. I buried my face in his neck and when I opened my eyes, I was inside my own ribcage, a scuba diver in clear physiological fluid. I took my flashlight through the water, scanning the web of bones, looking for my old fractures, trying to count them, but I could not do math. Neither could I drive, running my car over every curb, crashing a hundred times while my mother screamed in the front seat. The X-rays came in the mail. I had three broken ribs. The man and I were at a party, curled on the hardwood floor in each other's laps. I felt the warmth of his lips on my ear as he whispered, "why are you being so unkind to me." In this dream, everyone knew everything about us, especially the sins. Nobody would help me.

In This Dream I Call 911

And
nobody
picks
up.

Rate Your Pain:

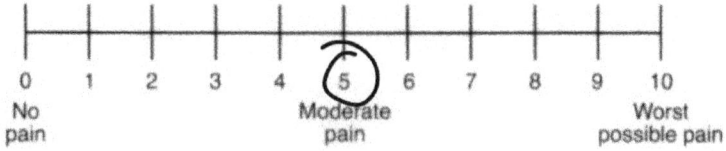

0	1	2	3	4	⑤	6	7	8	9	10
No pain					Moderate pain					Worst possible pain

Cracked asphalt
1500hours

Mid August
Burning off

NO Callus

Hurt Most

He looked me in the eye and begged me to
Let him die

As if that were in my power. The bullet he had meant
For his heart had instead spun through his spleen—

I have wanted to die for fifty years
He says, *ever since my first wife died*

The second wife is quiet in the waiting room
Please just let me die—

But the surgeon rolled him to the operating room,
Stuck a tube down his throat,

Slit his large belly,
Pulled out the ruined organ,

And made him live.

Postscript

That night I called that man I loved
Who also often wanted to die
I made him hold onto me
But didn't have the courage to ask my expert
If you have a death wish and find a gun in your hand
Why would you trust the inexact science of
Daring a bullet to hit your heart?

Psalm for My Body

There are contracts between genealogy and fate that I was not present to sign. Somehow I must come to terms with the things inside me that don't sit flush. That I was not constructed with a level in hand. I put my palm to my lips and try to think about the warmth in terms of sun-hours and tablespoons of chili. I am still learning to pray in the cathedral of my body, lighting candles not to burn it down, but to honor the women who split themselves to get to me.

I Dreamt My Own Evisceration

And kept apologizing. I held pressure to the stranger's ankle cut in the ballroom and kept my gown on to hide my abdomen's deep shred. I threw stitch after stitch in the woman's small tear, closing it, ignoring the strips of flesh dangling from my stomach looking like ground meat. I kept picking up bodies, stitching, fixing, hopping red puddles in formalwear amidst a flock of tuxedos, trying to repair every soon-to-be scar as my intestines slid out of my annihilated muscles. Nobody would help me.

Rate Your Pain:

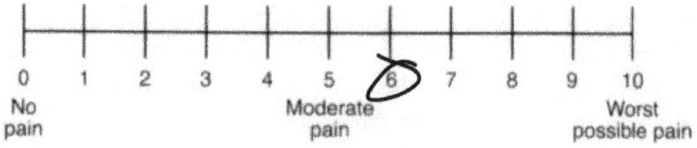

```
   |—|—|—|—|—|—|—|—|—|—|
   0   1   2   3   4   5  (6)  7   8   9   10
   No                 Moderate            Worst
   pain                  pain         possible pain
```

Lazy fascia
Colorless tracer the suffusing
Himalayas   Something shorter

Hills   boil   over

Fizzing back and around like Buzzards
         Waiting for   meat

The Angel in the Lion's Den

The angel flies down and the lion's jaws don't bite, every mouth stuck shut in gentle whiskering, sharp teeth sheathed, those first hours of warmth, the Daniel warmth, the fur on him weak, a warm slip, his warm small hands and his warm small breath. The lions sleep at night for the first time with their new Daniel, who makes them hungry but docile. A pride of sleeping breath floating out of the den, curling into Media, his small warm breath sweet smelling; the hunger of him seeps into the air. The Daniel kneels restless, making small warm sounds while the lions bat at the bones, the guilt settles heavy on him, with cubs and mothers snuffling at his head gently, learning their Daniel, mothers without milk today.

Daniel in the Lion's Den

The angel takes pity on the lions, comes back, unseals the jaws, and the lions stare softly, the Daniel dares not move, the mothers come nuzzle him to sleep, the best cure for hunger they know. This is the story of a Daniel who stays, whom God smiles on and kings leave to die, who is warm and soft and good, who learns to suck marrow after the lions dismantle their infidels. This Daniel, the one who stays, sleeps on the bellies of the lions. They eat apart at first and then together, him just the marrow, though the mothers try to give him more. The small warm Daniel grows his own wispy fur all over his tiny body, upon which the cubs curl after noon. The Daniel pleads his small sounds and shuffles through the carcasses, looking for marrow, combs and frets with the manes, and the mothers keep thinking the Daniel will grow, but he stays their cub.

The Boneheap in the Lion's Den

So the Daniel sucks the marrow and his breath smells sweet and the lions lay their paws upon him, their claws sheathed, and he falls under their weight and they wait for him to get up and he slowly gets up while they lick and tousle him and the cubs grow knowing only the time with the Daniel and they know the Daniel does not grow bigger, just darker around the face and smaller in the eyes and he stops making so many sounds and he stops kneeling on his little legs and he starts eating the bloody morsels, once Chosen People, and he stays up through the dark for many cubs and many nights and many infidels until finally he falls asleep, one last time, the boneheap.

What TV Gets Wrong

When the patient has
Disseminated
Intravascular
Coagulopathy
They do not have a delicate nosebleed,
They turn purple and drizzle
And you will not save them.

There Is a Bad Kind of Miracle

Remember the man, the one who wanted to die, with two wives, his enormous old body a cage he could not sing through? I kept some secrets. I apologize. Spleens are small. It would have been easier to shoot the large bowel, the span of liver, even a lung, but instead the spleen caught the bullet. Spleens love to bleed, often need to be pulled out of bodies and thrown away, unlike a kidney we would have cradled, or a liver we would have tenderly patched, he shot his fucking spleen, not the intended heart. Both would have granted him eventual death, but the spleen is a modest, inessential bundle of vessels that would seep slow, take its time to kill him, as if he hadn't been hurting long enough.

Rate Your Pain:

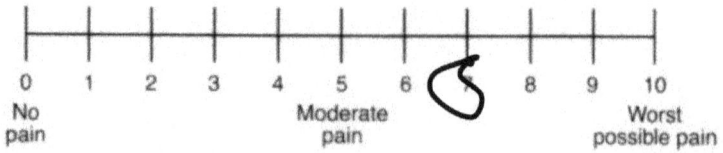

```
|--+--+--+--+--+--+--+(7)--+--+--|
0   1   2   3   4   5   6   7   8   9   10
No              Moderate          Worst
pain              pain          possible pain
```

lightning arcing in a wayward spin

peregrine Falcon
wing span until   the

ACDC Blast
singeing   feathers

skyscream falling
   hot   dead   meat

For the John Doe We Sliced Open

And buried without a name on the stone
Whose life is a screen door still
Hanging off the hinges
Waiting for you to walk back through it?

Bleeding Experiments

I. Prisoner of War (POW)

Some nights the pain has a gun
to my head
and makes me recite *dulce et decorum est*
pro patria mori
until I almost believe it.

Dulce et decorum
        From Wilfred Owen,
        Meaning sweet and fitting
                Sweet as in: the red coating on ibuprofen
                Left in your cheek too long
                Fitting as in: this is something you deserve

Pro patria
        From the Latin, meaning
        For my mother, Patricia, from whom all the pain
        Seems to have come
        Despite her lifetime of love as apology
        I scour my genes
        Speculate
        As in: a person who makes a risky investment
                Or goes out trying to find gold
                With nothing but a pickaxe

Mori
        As in: more
                As in: the story is not finished
Mori
        As in: dead

II. Fucked Up Beyond All Recognition (FUBAR)

You accept the pain you think you deserve
The rest gets bailed out of you
By whoever is nearby
Whether that is a surgeon
      As in: the surgeons who filled rags with blood and shit
      Since the bullet had sliced the bowel
      As in: a parent
      Writing poems about heroin relapse
      Because they keep happening
      Over and over
      He uses the words "YET ANOTHER"
           As in: a continuous series

Heroin annihilates pain annihilates imagination
      Cannot imagine
      As in: what it feels like to do heroin, according to
      My hollowed out patients whose veins are FUBAR

Key words "beyond all"
      Hour sixteen unseams my body
      Does not believe in
      Sweet or sleep or sex anymore

I stalk down endless white hallways
And imagine tripping
Falling flat forward
No nasal bones perforating brain
Because just as I hit the floor
My whole body dissolves
And disappears into the
Floor unseen beyond all recognition

III. Absent Without Leave (AWOL)

Pain is the coal miner, black lunged, wry smile,
Giving you a wink as he walks back
Underground
        As in: the emergency room
        Outside which the news crews hold court
        Using our doors as a backdrop
        For the story about 11 shootings and 7 homicides in 1 night

Pain is the paring knife
In your grandmother's hands as she slowly turns the apple
Making fragile and friable
That which was whole and strong
        As in: the man sitting in a nurse's desk chair
        Holding gauze to his own shoulder
        So his bullet wound
        Does not drip
        All over the floor

IV: Missing in Action (MIA)

IV: as in: intravenous
    As in: the anesthesiologist screaming
    With shaking hands
    In the operating room
    Because he cannot
    Get anything into the patient's veins
    Because they are collapsed
        As in: the brother of our
        Braindead ICU patient
        Crumpling to the floor
            As in: where the same brother
            Later threw trashcans at other families
            In the waiting room

Missing
    As in: where does the pain go when it is not hurting you?

Rate Your Pain:

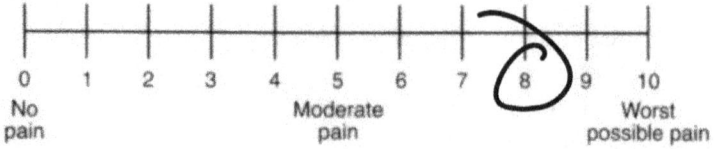

0 1 2 3 4 5 6 7 8 9 10
No pain

Moderate pain

Worst possible pain

dissolving
spattered
fissure
blown
pulp
oozing
acing
anatomic

A Foal a Key and Sobs

You can copy a key for 35 cents at my local hardware store even if it says no copies but when you copy keys they fit worse in the door I don't know much of doors or much of keys but my old life taught me plenty about foals like that foals stand minutes after birth run days later you don't have to keep foals tied up only keep their mothers on a line and the baby will follow her anywhere the key to sobbing is do it in the shower if not you can cry on the floor that's okay too because you can use your feet to block the door so nobody will come inside by accident and see your fetal body mushed into the carpet like you owed it a favor if you're in bed when you sob make sure to keep your face to the ceiling else your sinuses will fill unevenly when you lay back know that the tears will puddle in your ears and if you happen to be in an emergency room when this happens don't scare everyone by screaming at the sensation of the warm liquid in your ears mistaking it for blood.

I Dreamed I Broke My Fibula

The whole head snapped off as I turned around
And though proven on X-ray,
Even my mother told me
The pain was in my head,
That there was work to be done
And I was malingering
In multiples pieces
I found a hospital
Like the one where I lost my first patient
And begged for pain medicine
Begged for a cast
Begged for crutches
Begged
But nobody would
Help me.

Delusion

One night in St. Louis the machinegun fire is so regular I pretend it is thunder. I stand in my kitchen waiting as a child, safe somewhere in Maryland, waits at the edge of a pool during a storm. I count off "one-one-thousand, two-one-thousand..." as if the seconds between shots, if divided by five, tell me how many miles away the lightning is, and how close it is to destroying me.

"Lost on You" – LP

There's a song that goes
"Hold me like you've never lost your patience"
But in my head I sing
"Hold me like you've never lost a patient"

Precious Metals

His little body an apostrophe
Little boy body pierced with hot metal
Small metal small body
Speculation then stillness
Rooms that are never dark suddenly still
His body a little bump under the sheet
Quiet hands pass around metal
Ask metal questions
Call for bags of red liquid metal
The panic in my throat metal
A feeling cuffed phantom around wrists
Teeming with red metal
The minutes metal
The relief of the metal bed rails put up
His heart pumping metal
The new knights from next-door
Wheel to the children's hospital
A comma thank God not a period

Rate Your Pain:

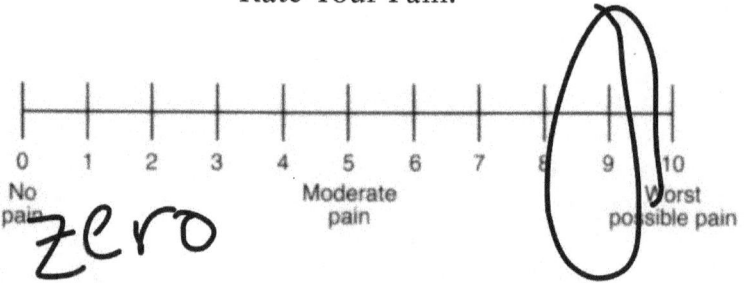

```
    0   1   2   3   4   5   6   7   8   9  10
    No              Moderate            Worst
    pain              pain          possible pain
```

zero
speed

everest french
pressure

blackhole
exhaustion

locomotive

Munchausen

Fire and Ice

I am feeling argumentative again. The politicians, the news anchors, the men wearing Remington shirts, I want to stand before them. I want to say something about gunfire, about how they wouldn't call it that if they saw bullets when I see them, cold, sticky, still. I would make some grandiose reference to Frost, say something about death nobody had ever said before, heat making bodies cold, fire and ice, but I can't stop thinking about the chilled muzzle of a gun, my body blasting with warm chemicals and sweat. Gunfire. I still remember the pitifully small, misshapen bullet we pulled from a man's bladder, its quiet ping like a windchime.

Soon

nobody will   remember   my   name

when they think

of their dead

child.

In Defense of the ICD System

Listen, we were trying to keep this unsaid, but you're leaving us without choices. We are not the icy fools you make us out to be. How have you not yet figured this out: it is easier to talk about the patients in numbers and single letters, to reduce everything from a broken pelvis to homelessness down to an ICD-10 code. Think just for a second about *us*, we don't have time to write this many goddamn poems. You can't expect us to live it all *de novo*, to sit by the chart and write

Here lies
The child.
What's left of him.
What the molten asphalt
Didn't burn away
When he was crushed
By the county-owned steamroller,
What remains after
The fifty times
We have pressed
Our scalpels into him,
Peeling him away
Gram by gram,
Applying salves and chemicals
In a salvage mission.

We don't want to write that poem, to be tasked with titling it, to have to write it and then start reducing the five hundred lines of our shock and continuous grief so it will fit on the page. When you start writing that poem you won't stop, not for hours, and there are 26 patients on your service today. It is necessary to create limits, to not start the poems in the first place, for the sake of productivity. We will put instead "W31.9: contact with unspecified machinery," and be done with it.

For Owners of a Ribcage

When you find yourself beneath a steamroller you will burst
Like a Christmas ornament
Under a boot.

Rate Your Pain:

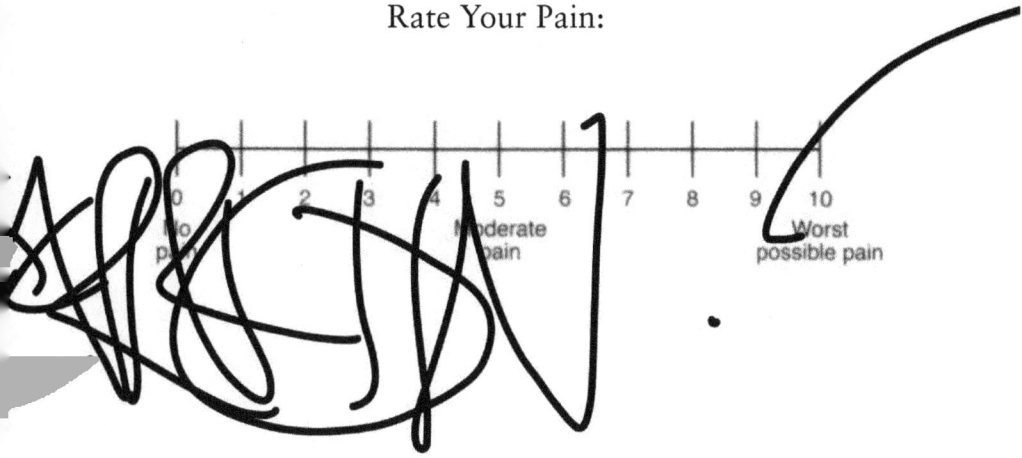

0   1   2   3   4   5   6   7   8   9   10
No   Moderate   Worst
pain   pain   possible pain

*carrion

Ten

"You know my student,
the 4th grader you met,
she
was
shot
and
killed
this
summer."

What It's Like Off Shift

Her ghost was in my bed again last night.
I sang a lullaby, I rocked, she breathed.
I held her to me, and she stayed awhile.

Trauma Surgeon Ars Poetica

This morning a robin collides with the glass windows of our sunroom. It flies into three panes, then four, then the same one many times, looking for different skies, trying to escape the day. With each thump I think, "this is the sort of thing poets write about, those poets who know how to hide the word death inside of a songbird," but I don't know how to talk about blood without speaking the scarlet spatter of it. I say nothing to the red-brown bird, the reflection of the sky's blue face veined with branches, the feathers so light they seem to shirk the responsibility of falling, the dull thunk ringing in the house, the morning so quiet it becomes prayer, the lined triangle of yellow beak, the black moon of the eye intent on its mirage. I cannot write that poem. I am still thinking about blood. When I see the robin throw itself at the window a fifth, sixth, seventh time, I open the door, I wave my arms, I chase it away.

Notes

"Red"

"I know a man who took a double ax
And went alone against a grove of trees;
But his heart failing him, he dropped the ax
And ran for shelter quoting Matthew Arnold:
'Nature is cruel, man is sick of blood'"
—Robert Frost, "New Hampshire"

"Massive Transfusion Protocol"

An adult male's body contains on average 5 liters of blood.
We transfused one of my trauma patients about 250 units of
donated red blood cells, plasma, and platelets in a single night.
A blood bag contains about 450ml of product, so

$$\frac{\left(250 bags \times 0.45\frac{ml}{bag}\right)}{5000\frac{ml}{person}} \approx 22.5 \text{ people's worth of blood.}$$

"That Smell"

The American College of Surgeons (ACS) STOP THE BLEED®
program is part of a federal initiative to train civilians to
perform lifesaving maneuvers to stop fatal bleeding. I helped
teach this course while working with The T, a grassroots
antiviolence and social justice nonprofit in St. Louis.

"Eavesdropping on the Dead"

This poem is dedicated to Omar Almadani and his family.
Zaeem is the Arabic word for patriarch.
"Allah ateyk alf afyeeh" translates to, "May God give you well-
being in every aspect of your life."

"The Lies"
   The truth: this patient lived. Her daughters never came to visit.
   She left our hospital disfigured with scars, alive. I think about
   her all the time.

"And Your Daughters Shall Prophecy"
   From *The King James Bible*, Acts 2:17

"Caveat to Moratorium"
   According to a 2021 study, female surgeons are about twice
   as likely to have major pregnancy complications as their non-
   surgeon peers. One of my mentors, whose twins died at 20
   weeks gestation while their mother was on call, is among them.
   Rangel EL, Castillo-Angeles M, Easter SR, Atkinson RB, Gosain
   A, Hu YY, Cooper Z, Dey T, Kim E. "Incidence of Infertility
   and Pregnancy Complications in US Female Surgeons."
   JAMA Surg. 2021 Oct 1;156(10):905-915. doi: 10.1001/
   jamasurg.2021.3301. Erratum in: JAMA Surg. 2021 Oct
   1;156(10):991. PMID: 34319353; PMCID: PMC9382914.

"Post Script"
   Between 2010 and 2020, 102,774 American men over the age
   of 65 died via firearm injury. Of those deaths, 89.6% were
   suicides. Centers for Disease Control and Prevention, National
   Centers for Injury Prevention and Control. Web-based Injury
   Statistics Query and Reporting System (WISQARS) [online].
   (2005) {2022 11 13}. Available from: www.cdc.gov/injury/
   wisqars

"The Angel in the Lion's Den"
   From *The King James Bible*, Daniel 6:16- Daniel 6:23

"What TV Gets Wrong"
   From LP's "Lost on You," Vagrant Records, 2015

"Bleeding Experiments: I. Prisoner of War (POW)"
From Wilfred Owen's "Dulce et Decorum Est," Viking Press,
1921

"Bleeding Experiments: II. Fucked Up Beyond All Recognition (FUBAR)"
From "Yet Another Heroin Relapse" by Richard W. Downing.

"A Foal a Key and Sobs"
Title extracted from the Robert Frost title, "A Fountain, A
Bottle, A Donkey's Ears and Some Books."

"Precious Metals"
*A Violent Summer for St. Louis Children Leaves Everyone
Grasping for Answers.* (2019, September 26). STLPR. https://
news.stlpublicradio.org/government-politics-issues/2019-09-26/
a-violent-summer-for-st-louis-children-leaves-everyone-grasping-
for-answers

"In Defense of the ICD System"
For billing and research purposes, hospitals in the United States
use the tenth iteration of the International Diagnosis Code
(ICD) System. This system assigns each malady a series of
numbers, letters, and decimals to specify the condition.

"Ten"
This poem is dedicated to Nyla Banks, my friend's former
student, who was murdered just after I moved out of St. Louis.
Her case remains unsolved.
*"Who Could Be This Heartless?": 10-Year-Old Girl and Her
Parents Found Brutally Murdered in Their St. Louis Apartment.*
(2019, August 28). Oxygen Official Site. https://www.oxygen.
com/crime-time/nyla-banks-antoinette-banks-and-gene-watson-
iii-found-murdered-in-st-louis-apartment

Acknowledgments

I am grateful to the editors of the following publications for publishing my poems, some in different versions:

Auxocardia, "What It's Like Off Shift"

Journal of the American Medical Association, "Trauma Surgeon Ars Poetica"

Op Med: Voices from the Doximity Network, "Precious Metals"

Snapdragon: A Journal of Art and Healing, "In Defense of the ICD System"

Tendon Magazine, "Hurting Instructions," "Ten" [as "Losing Her"], "I Dreamed I Coughed Up My Spine" [as "New Dreams"]

Tofu Ink, "The Body Only Speaks Her Own Language," "Psalm for My Body"

I would like to thank my parents and siblings for packing my bags with love. Thank you to my friends Lia, Suraj, Mark, and Margaux.

I owe much of this book to my former teachers and writing mentors, including Maggie Spak, Nathaniel Rosenthalis, and Dr. Jennifer Arch. Thank you to Tom Lombardo for selecting my manuscript and for helping me bring it into its final form. Thank you to Kevin Watson and Press 53 for all their support.

Finally, thank you to Dr. Bochicchio and Kelly Bochicchio for hiring me onto your "Bleeding Experiment" those many years ago.

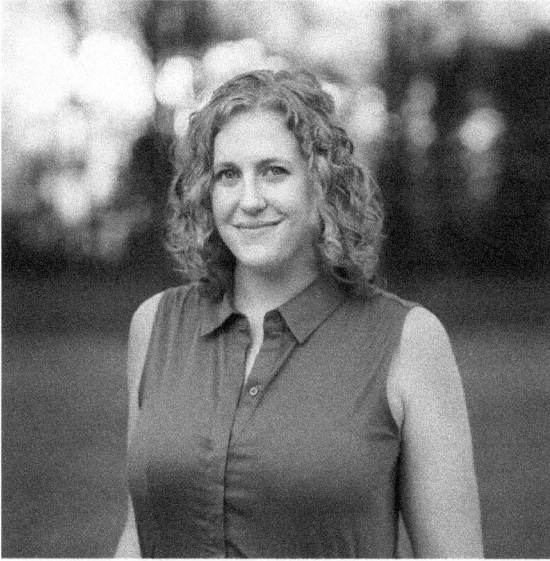

Maya J. Sorini is a poet, performer, and medical student from Rockville, Maryland. She received her B.A. in Chemistry from Washington University in St. Louis while engaging in clinical trauma surgery research. After finishing her undergraduate degree, Maya pursued a Master of Science in Narrative Medicine at Columbia University. She is currently pursuing a Doctor of Medicine at Hackensack Meridian School of Medicine and lives in Bergen County, New Jersey, with her grandmother. The poems in this collection are largely based on Maya's experiences working with trauma patients in St. Louis.